The Art of Food Freedom
Breaking Bad Eating Habits for a Balanced Life

Norman Phillip Fisher

Table of Contents

Food is an important part of a balanced diet.

— Fran Lebowitz

Chapter 1. Introduction

Welcome to "The Art of Food Freedom: Breaking Bad Eating Habits for a Balanced Life," where you pave the way towards a wholesome and vibrant life! In this Special Report, you'll discover how to break free of the invisible chains of bad eating habits and foster a joyous, loving relationship with food. No longer will you battle with guilt or confusion; instead, embark on a journey of liberation, learning to savor food while maintaining a balanced, healthy lifestyle. Our expert advice, practical strategies, and inspiring success stories will not only change your approach towards nutrition but also transform your life in profound ways. You're just one step away from breaking those barriers to food freedom. Are you ready to make the transformation? This report is your key. Welcome aboard!

Chapter 2. Understanding Our Relationship with Food

To understand our relationship with food, it is crucial to delve deeper into the fundamentals of how we perceive food, its importance in our life, and the psychological factors that play a role. This comprehensive exploration of the human-food connection will offer an extensive understanding, shedding light on the reason why changing eating habits is a complex, multifaceted challenge.

2.1. The Complexity of Human and Food Interactions

Our relationship with food is not just about the consumption of nutrients. Every individual experiences food differently. For some, it is a source of comfort, while for others, it is merely a necessity. The way we interact with food gets influenced by an assortment of factors, including culture, family traditions, taste preferences, emotional states, lifestyle, and our body's nutritional needs. This rich tapestry of influences can make our relationship with food more convoluted than it often appears.

Firstly, cultural influences and family traditions hold a significant influence over dietary choices. The types of food we prefer, how we prepare them, and even how we consume them has strong roots in our cultural background, and these traditions are passed through generations, shaping our relationship with food from a very early age.

Similarly, personal taste preferences also have a sway over the food choices we make. These preferences are not finalized at birth. Instead, they evolve over time, influenced by experiences, environment, and even the people we surround ourselves with.

Furthermore, our emotional states are greatly intertwined with our food intake. 'Emotional eating' is a very real phenomenon, where individuals turn towards food for comfort in times of stress, sadness, or even boredom. Understanding the role of emotions in our food choices can be a pivotal step in reforming our eating habits.

Simultaneously, our lifestyle and the pace at which we live also affect our relationship with food. In our fast-paced, convenience-oriented society, it is easy to prioritize speed and accessibility over health and nutrition. This, in turn, can lead to a lifestyle where meal prep and mindful eating take the backseat, and fast food and snacking take the forefront.

Lastly, our body's nutritional needs play a straightforward role in how we relate to food. This relationship can be distorted, though when these needs are overshadowed by the aforementioned factors, leading to a disconnect from our body's true signals of hunger and satiety.

2.2. Psychological Factors Impacting our Relationship with Food

Psychology plays a paramount role in our eating habits. Our mindset, attitudes, and unconscious biases can become significant determinants of how we perceive food.

One of the most prevalent psychological phenomena affecting our eating habits is the diet mentality, wherein food is viewed categorically as 'good' or 'bad.' This binary outlook can result in feelings of guilt when consuming purportedly 'bad' foods and an overly restrictive approach towards eating.

Moreover, societal pressures and norms also dictate our perceptions of food and body image. Constant exposure to unrealistic body standards and diet culture can affect our self-esteem and skew our relationship with food, leading to harmful behaviors such as incessant dieting, body dissatisfaction, and even eating disorders.

Psychologists also often mention the concept of 'food as a reward.' This refers to the conditioning process in which certain foods, usually high in sugar or fat, are offered as a reward, leading us to develop a positive association with such foods. Over time, these learned associations can result in overeating and preferring unhealthy foods, further compounding the issue of poor eating habits.

2.3. Understanding Our Personal Relationship With Food

Given the complexities and the deeply-rooted nature of our relationship with food, evaluating our personal interaction with food becomes an essential step towards making healthier eating decisions.

Self-observation, introspection, and awareness are key to recognizing and understanding the patterns of our eating behaviors. It is essential to be mindful of the 'whys' behind our food choices. This encompasses questioning the emotional, cultural, psychological, and physical factors compelling our eating habits.

One effective method is keeping a food diary — not so much for controlling calorie intake but to track eating patterns, types of food eaten, and emotional responses associated with food. This exhaustive record can provide insightful details about our eating habits which could be otherwise easily overlooked.

Another crucial aspect is understanding the difference between emotional hunger and physical hunger. It is practical to note and differentiate the signs associated with each form of hunger – for instance, emotional hunger usually comes on suddenly and urges the intake of specific comfort foods, while physical hunger is more gradual and open towards different food options.

In essence, if we aim for a healthy and balanced approach towards eating, it is vital that we thoroughly dissect and comprehend our intricate relationship with food. This wide-ranging exploration can equip us with the understanding to make conscious, mindful choices about what we eat, why we eat it, and how we can establish a more constructive relationship with food moving forward. This is the first step towards achieving food freedom and breaking the cycle of harmful eating habits.

Chapter 3. The Roots of Bad Eating Habits

Unhealthy eating habits have their roots tangled deep in our psyche, our environment, and our lifestyle. Many factors contribute to the formation of such detrimental habits. To fully confront and transform our eating behaviors, we must first trace them back to their origin - our past experiences, our psychological tendencies, our cultural background, and our current lifestyle.

3.1. The Influence of Childhood Experiences

One of the core origins of bad eating habits lies in our childhood experiences. Early habits surrounding food are significantly influenced by family customs, traditions, and attitudes. Often, they're shaped in the context of reward systems, such as offering sweets or desserts as a treat for good behavior, or forcing children to clean their plates. Over time, these experiences contribute to the foundation of our relationship with food, fostering attitudes that may lead to overeating, under-eating, or an unhealthy preoccupation with certain types of food.

3.2. The Role of Emotional Eating

Emotional eating is another significant factor contributing to negative food habits. People often turn to food for comfort during times of stress, loneliness, anxiety, or even boredom. This form of self-soothing can develop into a deep-seated habit, creating a cycle where emotional distress leads to overeating, followed by feelings of guilt and even more stress, resulting in further overindulgence. Although these temporary comforts might seem effective at the moment, they often lead to long-term physical and psychological health issues.

3.3. Culture and Society: Crucial Determinants

Our culture and society also play a significant role in shaping our eating patterns. The societal norms, marketing strategies, and lack of access to healthy and nutritious foods greatly contribute to the development of unhealthy eating habits. Fast food advertisements and societal pressures to maintain certain body standards can greatly influence both our perception about food and our eating behaviors. The urge to fit into these societal norms often pushes individuals toward unhealthy dieting behaviors or binge eating.

3.4. Sedentary Lifestyles and Convenience Foods

With advancements in technology and changes in lifestyle, our dependency on convenience foods has skyrocketed. The modern world's fast-paced lifestyle often forces individuals to rely on processed, high-calorie foods lacking in nutritional value. Additionally, a sedentary lifestyle coupled with an abundance of readily available unhealthy food options sets a fertile ground for bad eating habits to take root and flourish.

3.5. Inadequate Nutritional Knowledge

A lack of understanding of nutrition is another root cause of unhealthy eating habits. Without adequate knowledge about the nutritional value of different foods, and what a balanced diet should include, it becomes difficult to make informed, healthy food choices. Let's not forget, making sense of food labels and dietary advice is a daunting task even for adults. Providing comprehensive nutritional education is a key strategy for paving the way to healthier eating habits.

Tracing the roots of unhealthy eating habits is an essential first step toward fostering food freedom. Recognizing that these habits are often complex and deep-seated helps to contextualize the struggle and resist the urge to self-blame. However, they are not indelible marks on our lives. Having understood the origins of these food behaviors, we can now move on to strategies that can help us break these patterns, which is the next focus of our journey.

Chapter 4. The Psychology Behind Food Choices

Our journey into investigating the psychology behind food choices begins with acknowledging a truth we often overlook: our food choices do not always align directly with our health goals. The intricate labyrinth of factors that sculpt our eating behaviors is bewildering, with inputs from our physiology, upbringing, emotions, environment, and even society at large.

4.1. Exploring the Psychological Factors

Arguably the most critical component in understanding the motivations behind our food choices are psychological factors. These elements include our emotions, stress levels, and habits.

Emotions have a stronger grip on our eating choices than most like to admit. We often find solace in comfort foods when we are sad, upset, or stressed, giving rise to emotional eating. Comfort foods are predominantly those high in fat, sugar, or both, as they help trigger the release of certain brain chemicals that make us feel better.

Stress, another emotional factor, plays a significant role in determining our eating habits. When stressed, our bodies release hormones that can increase our appetite or desire for high-calorie foods. It's no coincidence that during stress-filled times, we often seek solace in our favorite indulgence foods.

Simultaneously, our habits, cultivated over the years, significantly impact our food preferences. The recurring pattern of choosing certain foods over others shapes our taste palette and food choices as we age.

4.2. Social and Cultural Influences

Our cultures and societies influence these habits, making some choices seem natural or normal to us. Traditional cuisines and food habits, linked intrinsically with our emotions and memories, can be hard to change. For instance, if your family had a practice of enjoying sugary desserts after every dinner, you'd likely continue this tradition without questioning its impact on your health.

In many societies, food is often a symbol of love, celebration, or community. Holiday meals, birthday cakes, or community feasts are all deeply ingrained food patterns associated with happiness and belonging, which can sometimes lead to overeating or unhealthy food choices.

Moreover, peer pressure and societal standards can add a layer of complexity to our food choices. Often, people lean toward meals and dietary practices glorified by their social circles. These could range from trendy diets and detoxes to indulgent, excessive meals.

4.3. Food Marketing and Availability

In the modern world, food marketing and food availability significantly influence food choices. Supermarkets and online platforms make high-calorie, processed food readily available and attractive. It's a common experience to enter a supermarket intending to buy healthy food options and leaving with a trolley full of processed, high-sugar, or high-fat foods. This susceptivity is due to the strategic placement, branding, and promotions associated with unhealthy food options.

Food marketing isn't confined only to supermarkets. Most food advertisements on television, social media, or billboards glorify unhealthy food items, manipulating our choices sub-consciously.

4.4. Nutritional Knowledge and Food Attitudes

Finally, our knowledge about nutrition and our attitudes towards food influence our food choices. With access to the internet, information about various diets, food strategies, and nutritional advice is readily available. This information, however, can be conflicting or confusing, sometimes leading to unhealthy diets based on misinformation.

Despite the abundance of nutritional knowledge available, how much of this information translates into practice also depends on our attitude towards food. Attitudes such as 'I deserve this piece of cake after a hard day' or 'Healthy food doesn't taste good' are hurdles in the path of making healthy food choices.

Understanding these psychological, societal, and informational factors that impact our food choices is a crucial step towards changing them. By acknowledging the emotional, cultural, and cognitive aspects of our eating habits, we can pave the way towards healthier, more enlightened decision-making around food.

4.5. Conscious and Mindful Eating as a Solution

Conscious and mindful eating may be a viable solution to address the complex psychology of food choices. It involves savoring every bite of the food and being mentally present while we eat. It also means recognizing hunger signs and differentiating them from emotional cravings.

In conclusion, the psychology behind food choices is a complex phenomenon. It is a byproduct of a myriad of factors extending beyond the boundary of hunger and nutritional requirements.

However, with a clear understanding of these influences, it is possible to channel a positive mindset towards food and work towards breaking free from unhealthy eating patterns. Endeavoring to cultivate healthy psychological attitudes towards food choice can contribute significantly to the overall quality of our lives and well-being.

Chapter 5. Your Body, Your Temple: The Importance of Good Nutrition

The human body, an intricate and magnificent creation of nature's artistry, is an embodiment of extraordinary complexity yet harmonious synchronicity. It houses systems that perform distinct functions yet converge towards maintaining a delicate equilibrium. Thus, to comprehend the importance of nutrition, it is essential to understand first the nature and structure of this complex architecture we call the body.

5.1. The Cellular Connection

On the most minute level, the human body comprises trillions of cells, each holding a universe within itself, performing vital biochemical processes. Nutrition directly influences these microcosmic entities. Cells harness energy from the food we consume and utilize it for everyday bodily functions. It's somewhat like fine-tuning your vehicle with the right fuel; it can surely run on low-quality gasoline, but for a smooth, efficient ride, premium fuel is necessary. Similarly, cells work best when supplied with nutrients of optimal quality.

5.2. An Ode to Our Organs

Consider your body as a grand orchestra, with each organ playing a significant yet distinct role. Your heart maintains the rhythm of life, your lungs lend the breath to that rhythm, kidneys diligently perform the task of detoxification, your brain – the prodigious maestro, controls and coordinates all these operations. This melodious harmony thrives on nutritional notes. A balanced diet reinforces their performances, preserving the orchestra's lifetime and quality of music.

5.3. The Food-Fuel Analogy

To illuminate the concept, consider food as fuel. If we treat our bodies like a machine, nutrition becomes the fuel that keeps us running. But, not all fuels are created equal. Some provide a clean, efficient burn, while others might leave behind harmful residues, leading to adverse effects like weight gain, lethargy, or worse, chronic conditions. The quality of fuel closely parallels the health and efficiency of the machine. Therefore, the food we eat and the nutrients it offers are a determinant of our overall health and vitality.

5.4. The Role of Macronutrients and Micronutrients

Nutrition is usually dissected into two subcategories: macronutrients and micronutrients. Macronutrients, comprised of carbohydrates, proteins, and fats, are energy-providing nutritional components that our bodies need in large amounts. Their primary role is to furnish energy, a vital currency for all our physiological functions.

On the other side of the nutrition spectrum reside micronutrients – vitamins and minerals. While required only in minor amounts, these dynamic warriors wear multiple hats. They act as catalysts in essential biochemical reactions, support the immune system, maintain bone health, boost cellular health, and promote adequate growth and development.

5.5. The Art of Balance

Balance is the essence of nutrition. An ideal harmony of macronutrients and micronutrients yields a balanced diet paving the way towards wholesome health. A leaning towards any one kind of nutrient can result in malnourishment, leading to a myriad of health issues.

5.6. Essential Nutrition Throughout Life Stages

Our nutritional requirements fluctuate throughout different life stages. From infancy through old age, adequate nutrition remains a constant prerequisite but varies in constituents and proportions. For instance, an adolescent might require higher protein nutrition to aid in their speedy growth, while an elderly individual might need more vitamins and minerals to bolster immunity and maintain vitality.

5.7. The Power of Prevention Through Nutrition

Besides influencing our daily physiological functions, nutrition holds the capacity to prevent several chronic diseases. By managing body weight and providing the nutrients required for the body to function effectively, a well-balanced diet reduces the risk of diseases like obesity, heart disease, diabetes, and some types of cancer. This preventive power of nutrition can't be overstated.

5.8. The Path to Mind-Body Wellness

Food's sphere of influence extends beyond the physical realm, leaving prominent imprints on mental health as well. A diet rich in essential nutrients helps stabilize moods, improve clarity, boost memory, and even limit the risk of mental health conditions like depression and anxiety.

Hence, the expression 'Your Body, Your Temple' is a profound reminder that the body is the sacred abode of your soul, demanding mindful nourishment and care. The importance of good nutrition cannot be overstressed, but it is vital to approach it with a mindset of reverence and respect for distinguishing its full potential. Armed with this knowledge, you stand at the threshold of a revolutionary journey towards a more vibrant and wholesome life.

Remember, the journey of a thousand miles begins with a single step. Treat your 'temple' with adoration, feed it with love and patience, and witness the magic transformation that ensues. Welcome to a healthier, happier you!

Chapter 6. Breaking the Cycle: Strategies to Overcome Bad Eating Habits

In our journey towards food freedom, once we acknowledge the unwholesome relationship we have established with our plates, it becomes essential to understand how to break this unhappy bond. Armed with these insights, knowledge, and conscious awareness, we can begin to replace destructive behaviors with healthier habits. This pivotal phase of transition, although challenging, serves as the primary agent for change, breaking the cycle and ushering in a new era of balance and harmony with food.

6.1. Understanding Trigger Foods

Trigger foods, those that either cause physical discomfort or provoke emotional turmoil such as cravings or binge-eating, can be outstandingly difficult to manage. Many individuals have at least a few foods that seem nearly impossible to eat in moderation. These could range from chips and candy to cheese and beer.

Identifying your trigger foods is crucial. Try to analyze your eating patterns and notice the foods that you consistently overeat, leaving you engulfed in guilt or physical discomfort afterward. If any such foods exist, it might be useful to maintain a 'food and mood' journal, recording not only what and when you eat but also noting the accompanying emotions and physical sensations.

Once you have identified these triggers, it could be beneficial to avoid them initially while you are trying to establish healthier habits. After you're more firmly grounded in your new, balanced relationship with food, you might consider reintroducing these items in a regulated manner.

6.2. The Art of Meal Planning

Meal planning is one of the most effective strategies to combat bad eating habits. It promotes mindful eating, encourages a well-rounded diet, and alleviates the stress of daily meal decisions.

Creating a weekly or monthly meal plan requires time and effort, but the benefits are copious. Start by choosing a variety of foods from each food group, ensuring a balanced intake of proteins, carbohydrates, fats, vitamins, and minerals. Then, write down the meals for the week, including breakfasts, lunches, dinners, and snacks.

Planning meals ahead of time can help lessen impulsive food choices and overeating. It allows for careful portion control and ensures that you have the necessary ingredients to prepare wholesome meals every day. Be sure not to fill your plan with exceedingly complicated recipes. Simple, nutritious meals are as beneficial, if not more.

To support your meal planning, consider meal prepping. It involves creating, cooking, and storing meals or meal components in advance. This strategy can save you time and further abate the urge to resort to unhealthy food options during busy workdays.

6.3. Transforming Your Food Environment

Upgrading your food environment is an instrumental factor in transforming eating habits. Start by purging your kitchen of unhealthy options. Keeping these comfort foods out of your immediate sight can dramatically lessen their temptation. Instead, stock your pantry and refrigerator with healthy, nutritious choices such as fruits, vegetables, lean proteins, and whole grains.

Remember, many eating habits are born out of convenience. If you have pre-cut fruits and vegetables ready to snack on, you're far less likely to reach for that bag of chips. Additionally, setting up your environment for mindful eating, like having a dedicated dining space free of distractions, can facilitate a conscious and relaxed eating experience.

6.4. Harnessing the Power of Mindful Eating

Mindful eating is a practice that cultivates a heightened awareness of the sensory pleasures of eating, your emotional cues, and physical hunger and satiety signals. It can assist in overcoming emotional eating and prevent mindless snacking.

To practice mindful eating, start by chewing your food slowly and savoring every mouthful. Dedicate yourself totally to the eating experience, eliminating distractions such as television or smartphones. Listen to your body's signs of hunger and fullness, understanding that it's okay to leave food on the plate when you're full.

Incorporating mindful eating into your daily routine is a gradual process. It's not about achieving perfection but fostering an improving relationship with food.

6.5. Enlisting Social Support

A journey of transformation is much more manageable when not undertaken alone. Enlisting social support can provide emotional reinforcement, keep you accountable, and motivate you to persist.

Seek out friends, family, professional counselors, or support groups who understand and respect your journey towards food freedom. Sharing your struggles and victories with like-minded individuals can fortify your resolve and provide a sense of belonging during difficult times.

To summarize, breaking the cycle of bad eating habits is no small feat. It demands introspection, determination, patience, and consistency. However, by understanding your triggers, planning your meals, transforming your food environment, practicing mindful eating, and enlisting the support of others, you are setting the stage for a successful transition towards a healthier, more balanced relationship with food. This journey may appear daunting, but remember, every small change you make brings you closer to your goal of food freedom.

Chapter 7. Practical Tips for Mindful Eating

Entering the realm of mindful eating means awakening to the stunning reality of our food - its vibrant colors, its tantalizing aromas, its texture in our mouths, and the nourishment it provides. By grounding ourselves in the present moment as we eat, we position ourselves not only to derive more pleasure and satisfaction from our meals but also to make wiser decisions regarding our food choices. Practicing mindful eating is a vibrant dance that frees us from automatic, habitual responses and opens us toward the possibility.

7.1. Becoming Aware of Your Hunger

The first step to mindful eating involves distinguishing between physical hunger, and mind hunger or emotional hunger. Physical hunger is the biological imperative signaling us to replenish nutrients, while emotional or mind hunger is triggered by emotional needs. Stress, boredom, loneliness, anger, or grief can create a false sense of hunger; we feel an urge to eat without feeling physical hunger. To distinguish, when the urge to eat arises, ask yourself: "Am I genuinely physically hungry or am I responding to an emotional need or mindless habit?" This self-questioning will help you realize whether you are eating in response to physical hunger or if this hunger is purely emotional. Moreover, pay attention to where in your body you feel hunger. Physical hunger can be felt in the stomach while emotional hunger can be commonly experienced in the heart or the head.

7.2. Eating Slowly

Eating slowly is one of the simplest yet most powerful practices of mindful eating. We often forget that digestion begins in the mouth, where enzymes in our saliva begin the process of breaking down food particles. By taking the time to chew thoroughly, we not only aid digestion and absorption but also give our brains the time they need to register feelings of fullness. Plus, we give ourselves more of an opportunity to savor each mouthful. Try to stretch your meals to 20-30 minutes, take smaller bites, and chew each mouthful 20-30 times to improve the experience and benefits from every meal.

7.3. Sensory Engagement

Imagine that you are a food critic, tasting a dish for the first time. Engage your five senses fully with each meal. Look at your food, holding an inner conversation about its colors and physical features. Smell your food: the aroma contributes significantly to its flavor. As you eat, savor the taste, notice the textures highlighted by your palate and be sensitive to the sound of your food as you chew. This mindful observation can bring out the little details about the food that you may have overlooked before, enhancing your meal experience.

7.4. Be Present in the Moment

Remove distractions such as turning off the television, putting down your phone, and stepping away from your desk or computer. By eating without distractions, you allow yourself to be present in the moment and pay full attention to your food, let it be your primary focus. Notice the preparation, savor the flavors, appreciate the nutritious value, and express gratitude for the nourishing sources. Mindful eating isn't just about the food but about the overall experience.

7.5. Making Mindful Food Choices

We must remember, using mindfulness as a tool for a better relationship with food doesn't mean restricting certain foods. Instead, it's about making conscious food choices. Be aware of how different foods affect your body and mood. Noticing these subtle changes will motivate you toward naturally healthier food, such as fresh fruits, vegetables, lean proteins, and whole grains.

7.6. Mindful Eating Meditation

Incorporating a mindful eating form of meditation into your routine could be a beneficial tool. Such a meditation would involve deep, focused breathing techniques, bringing your total attention to the current moment and the food you're about to consume, acknowledging and appreciating the physical and emotional sensations related to consuming food. Such practices turn a simple meal into a nourishing experience for both the body and mind.

In conclusion, mindful eating is a powerful tool in our journey toward food freedom. It assists us in breaking free from our automatic, thoughtless responses towards food and encourages thoughtful engagement and thorough enjoyment. Through these practical steps, you can incorporate mindful eating into your daily routine, leading to a healthier, wholesome, and more balanced relationship with food. Enjoy the journey; it's yours to make.

Chapter 8. Foods to Love and Foods to Limit: A Comprehensive Guide

Kicking off this invigorating exploration, we dive straight into the ocean of nutritious choices, navigating the shores of the foods you should befriend and the ones you might want to keep at arm's length for a balanced eating routine. This chapter shall indeed equip you with a comprehensive guide, threading together the fabric of a rich, varied, and nourishing diet.

8.1. The Power of Whole Foods

Whole foods are Mother Nature's unrivaled gift, a treasure trove of vitamins, minerals, and other essential nutrients necessary for optimal body functioning. These wholesome additions to your diet are generally not processed or refined, thereby conserving their nutritional profile intact. Whole foods include fruits and vegetables, whole grains, lean proteins, and legumes. Revere these items as the mainstays of your culinary journey, filling your plate with a rainbow of colors, shapes, and flavors. They are the gateway to a healthier you, providing you with energy, strengthening your immune system, and potentially warding off various ailments.

8.2. The Rainbow on Your Plate: Fruits and Vegetables

A diet rich in fruits and vegetables can be considered the cornerstone of nutritional wisdom. These brightly colored plant beings are literally packed with an astounding array of nutrients, each carrying their own distinctive array of health benefits. Fruits like berries, apples, and pears are brimming with necessary vitamins and fiber, bolstering your digestive health and curbing hunger. Vegetables, particularly dark leafy greens like spinach, kale, and broccoli, contain a proliferation of essential minerals and antioxidants that bolster your body in multiple ways. These delicious, natural, and fiber-rich foods aid in everything from heart health to skin clarity, often imparting a wonderful glow, satiety, and overall wellbeing.

8.3. Harnessing the Power of Whole Grains

Whole grains are an often overlooked superfood, teeming with a host of essential nutrients. This category includes foods like oats, brown rice, barley, and quinoa. Heralded for their high fiber content, these wholesome grains aid in digestion and help maintain blood glucose levels. Moreover, their richness in B-vitamins and iron plays a crucial role in energy production and maintaining good nervous system function. Swapping your refined grains with these nutritional powerhouses can be a simple yet significant step towards a balanced diet.

8.4. Lean Proteins: Building Blocks of Your Body

Consuming a suitable amount of protein is fundamental to building and repairing tissues, producing enzymes, and bolstering the overall health of various body organs and systems. Lean proteins such as chicken, turkey, fish, and eggs, provide you with the necessary protein without the extra fat and calories. For plant-based enthusiasts, legumes (such as lentils and chickpeas), tofu, tempeh, and seitan make excellent protein sources.

8.5. Legumes: The Nutrient Powerhouses

Lentils, beans, chickpeas, and peas – these humble legumes may not seem like much, but they are really nutrient powerhouses. Rich in fiber, protein, and low in fat, they are an excellent addition to any diet. The incredible benefits of legumes include improved digestion, regulating sugar levels, aiding in weight control, and even reducing the risk of heart disease.

8.6. Foods to Limit: Walking the Tricky Terrain

Equally pivotal as the identification of nourishing foods, is the judicious knowledge of Foods to Limit. These may include overly processed foods, sugary foods, or those high in unhealthy fats. While they may be tempting and momentarily satisfying, they can potentially wreak havoc on your well-being over time. These include foods such as processed meats, snack foods, sugary drinks, and others, which we'll examine in detail shortly.

8.7. Triggering the Traps: Processed Foods

Processed foods have become a staple in many diets due to ease and accessibility. But the cost to your health can outweigh these simple benefits. These foods frequently contain high levels of sodium, which in surplus, can contribute to hypertension and heart disease. Furthermore, the processing can strip these foods of their original nutrients, offering little in return for your body's needs.

8.8. The Sugary Slip: Refined Sugars

Sugar may be sweet, but its effects on health are far from it. Refined sugars, found in soda, baked goods, and many packaged foods, can lead to obesity, type 2 diabetes, and heart disease. It is healthier to satiate your sweet cravings with natural sugars from fruits, vegetables, and whole grains.

8.9. Bad Fats: Saturated and Trans Fat

Hidden in many foods like processed meats, baked goods, and fried foods, unhealthy fats are a silent detriment to your health. High consumption of saturated and trans fats can lead to high cholesterol levels, heart disease, or stroke. Prioritize the inclusion of healthier fats found in foods like avocados, nuts, and seeds.

Embarking on this journey, it is important to remember that limiting does not mean eliminating altogether. The objective is to foster a balance and nurture a healthy, steadfast relationship with food. This comprehensive guide serves as an insightful preamble to equip you to make informed choices, setting the stage for a change that extends beyond wanting to look a certain way to cherishing how it makes you feel, inside and out.

Chapter 9. Boosting Your Willpower: Techniques and Daily Practices

In this essential piece of the transformative journey, we dive deep into effective methods and everyday practices to augment your willpower. The significance of willpower in breaking bad eating habits and fostering a balanced lifestyle cannot be overstated; it is your resilience in the face of tempting unhealthy choices, your discipline when consuming food thoughtfully, and your courage when embracing change.

9.1. Cultivating an Iron Will

Observing successful individuals across a myriad of disciplines makes it abundantly clear that willpower is not an innate characteristic that some are blessed with while others languish in its absence. Rather, it's much like a muscle that can and should be consistently trained for it to grow stronger. One of the most powerful ways to cultivate willpower is through discipline, which takes root in your day-to-day habits.

Begin by establishing a structured routine that, over time, will require less conscious effort to maintain. This might include a healthy sleep schedule, time allotted for meal planning and preparation, and regular physical activity. In the case of food habits specifically, it's crucial that your routine aligns with your goal of eating healthier, factoring in elements such as grocery shopping for wholesome ingredients or practicing mindful eating during each meal.

Another vital facet is working on your patience and tolerance, especially for discomfort. In the context of eating habits, discomfort could arise in situations where you're making a conscious choice to avoid junk food when the craving hits, or opting for smaller portions despite the desire to eat more. Rather than immediately succumbing to these discomforts, allow yourself to experience them, reminding yourself that they are temporary and on the other side lies the gratification of having made a healthier choice.

9.2. Building Resilience through Effective Stress Management

Stress, often an unwelcome companion in our busy lives, can significantly undermine willpower. Studies reveal a distinct correlation between elevated stress levels and unhealthy food choices. Consequently, learning how to manage stress effectively becomes a prerequisite for boosting willpower.

Firstly, find what soothes and rejuvenates you. For some, this may be meditation or yoga, while others may find solace in painting or a brisk walk in nature. Regularly scheduled breaks during the day to consciously unwind and practice these stress-relieving activities can make a substantial difference.

In addition to recreational activities, establish supportive relationships with individuals who understand and resonate with your journey towards food freedom. Support groups or health-loving friends can serve as a powerful buffer against stress, offering motivation, advice, and shared experiences.

9.3. Harnessing the Power of Meditation and Mindful Practice

Meditation is an incredibly potent tool for strengthening willpower. It fosters a heightened sense of self-awareness, important for both identifying negative eating habits and proactively changing them. In addition, meditation has been shown to reduce stress and anxiety, both of which are proven contributors to unhealthy food choices.

When we bring mindfulness into eating specifically, we alter our relationship with food drastically. It is the practice of paying full attention to the act of eating - savoring each bite, appreciating the flavors, and recognizing when you're full. Regular practice of mindful eating fosters an innate understanding of what, when, and how much your body truly needs to consume.

Potentially, you could start with a simple 5-minute meditation every morning, focusing on your breath and the sensations in your body. As you progress, steadily increase the duration and incorporate mindful eating techniques into your meal times. Filling your plate with vibrant, wholesome foods and appreciating the nourishment they provide can be a transformative meditation in itself.

9.4. Positive Reinforcement: Visualizing Success and rewarding Progress

Visualization is a powerful technique used by athletes and high achievers across sectors. In your journey towards food freedom, visualize yourself comfortably and confidently making healthier food choices. The human brain is incredibly receptive to imagery; visualizing your success can create neural pathways that make the journey seem less challenging and the goals more attainable.

As equally important is the power of rewards. Rewarding yourself (not with unhealthy food, of course!) occupies an essential place in fostering willpower. The principle of Positivity Bias, the brain's tendency to respond more robustly to positive stimuli, means that when a behavior is rewarded, it is more likely to be repeated. Consider rewarding your milestone achievements with experiences like a day at the spa, buying that book you've wanted to read, or even an adventurous weekend getaway.

9.5. Consistency: Your Biggest Ally

Lastly, remember that consistency over perfection is the mantra when it comes to building willpower. It's about repeated effort, no matter how small, and an unwavering commitment to your healthy eating habits. Much like a long-distance race, it's not about speed; it's about resilience and staying the course despite the hurdles you might encounter.

By fostering willpower, you're not merely switching to healthier eating habits but evolving into a version of yourself that can face a challenge with grace, whether it's related to food or any other facet of your life. By embracing these techniques and incorporating them into your daily routines, you'll find that food no longer controls you – you are the captain of your own ship, sailing confidently towards the horizon of health and wellness. The day where you truly experience the art of food freedom isn't just a dream; with willpower on your side, it's an impending reality.

Chapter 10. Success Stories: Inspirational Journeys of Food Freedom

Success stories possess an unmatched power to motivate and inspire. In this chapter, we'll explore the real-life journeys of individuals who diligently weathered their own storms, conquered their own mountains, and transformed their relationship with food. They emerged victorious with a renewed understanding of how food can serve them, not enslave them, creating a roadmap for others to follow, to break free from bad eating habits, and achieve their Food Freedom.

10.1. John: Turning to a Plant-Based Regime

John was an office worker, whose daily routine primarily involved sitting in front of his computer. Over time, his nutritional balance started to skew negatively due to a lack of physical activity and the consumption of unhealthy food.

John was stuck in a bad eating cycle. This led to ongoing health problems that included obesity, high blood pressure, and frequent lethargy. John realized he needed to take charge of his own health. His decision to adopt plant-based eating was a significant turning point in his life. Learning about the environmental impact of his food choices and the health benefits of a vegetarian diet, he started to change his life one veggie meal at a time.

His initial transition was challenging. There were doubts, setbacks, and missteps. Despite these difficulties, John persevered. He devoted himself to meal planning, learned about plant-based proteins, and found ways to make his new diet enjoyable. Now, over a year later, John's lost over 60 pounds, his medical parameters have stabilized and he reports feeling more energetic than ever before.

10.2. Linda: Overcoming Emotional Eating

As a single mother of two navigating a high-stress job, Linda's eating habits were inconsistent at best. Often, she'd resort to emotional eating and late-night snacking, seeking solace in food. She was locked in the cycle of guilt and binge eating, which negatively impacted her overall health and vitality.

Deciding to transform her relationship with food, Linda worked with a knowledgeable dietitian and therapist. Through therapy, she dug into her emotional triggers for overeating, while the dietitian guided her towards healthier food options and appropriate portion sizes.

After a year of hard work, she has successfully overcome her emotional eating habits. She has conquered her late-night cravings and replaced them with healthier alternatives. By understanding her triggers, she took control of her body's natural needs and maintained her food freedom, enjoying her meals without guilt or regret.

10.3. Michael: Breaking Free from Processed Foods

Once an avowed fan of fast food, Michael's health took a toll due to his reliance on these processed, unhealthy meals. Diagnosed with high cholesterol and a fatty liver, he realized he needed to reevaluate his food choices.

He vowed to break free from processed foods. Looking for solutions, he consulted with a nutritionist who guided him towards whole, nutritious foods. The idea was to gradually replace fast-food items with wholesome meals, using fruits, vegetables, lean proteins, and whole grains.

It was an uphill climb, but Michael remained committed. He had some slip-ups, but these became less frequent as his taste palate adapted to healthier flavors. A year into his journey, Michael's cholesterol level is now within a healthy range, and his liver enzymes have normalized significantly. His story motivates others to believe in the power of beneficial food changes.

These narratives of transformation offer hope, motivation, and a testament to human resilience. Each journey illustrates an individual take on food freedom, inspiring all of us to take control of our eating habits and reclaim our health. However, remember that everyone's journey is unique. What works for John, Linda or Michael, might look different for you, and that's okay. Always consult health professionals when in doubt and keep your unique health needs in mind when embarking on your journey towards food freedom.

Chapter 11. Maintaining the Balance: Sustaining Healthy Eating Habits for Life

Achieving a healthy relationship with food is undeniably a significant milestone. But the journey doesn't end here; maintaining this balance for the rest of your life is the ultimate goal. This chapter aims to provide you with comprehensive and detailed information on sustaining these good eating habits throughout your life. We'll delve into the psychology behind relapses, the importance of consistency, implementing sustainable lifestyle changes, as well as the role of forgiveness and patience in this lifelong journey towards food freedom.

11.1. Understanding the Anatomy of a Relapse

Studies suggest that reversion or relapse in healthy eating habits is common for various reasons such as stress, lack of a supportive network, or unsustainable diet plans. It's essential to evaluate and understand the triggers behind these relapses to avoid them in the future effectively.

Understanding the anatomy of a relapse involves three stages:

1. Emotional trigger: An emotional event, like stress, anxiety, or grief, often sparks a relapse. Recognizing and managing these emotional triggers is fundamental to prevention.

2. Thought process: The emotional trigger typically results in destructive thought patterns like over-generalization, perfectionism, or excessive self-criticism.

3. Behavioral response: This stage involves indulging in unhealthy eating habits as a response to the emotional trigger and destructive thought patterns.

Regularly practicing mindfulness can help identify these patterns as they occur, reducing the instances of unhealthy responses and, as a result, relapses.

11.2. The Role of Consistency

Once you've comprehended the mechanisms behind a relapse and the ways to stave it off, it's time to focus on the backbone of maintaining healthy eating habits: consistency. Merely establishing good habits isn't sufficient; persevering and sticking to them over the long haul is crucial. Here's some advice to nurture consistency:

- Create specific, measurable, achievable, relevant, and time-bound (SMART) goals that will encourage progress and keep you motivated.

- Don't sway with the winds of dietary trends. Instead, follow a balanced and flexible diet that suits you best.

- Start with small changes and gradually incorporate more significant changes into your lifestyle.

- Practice intentional eating until it becomes second nature.

11.3. Implementing Sustainable Changes

Sustainable changes lean towards moderate and balanced choices that fit seamlessly into your lifestyle rather than drastic, restrictive alterations that may feel like punishment. Doing so ensures that the changes are manageable and conducive to long-term implementation. Here are some ways to foster sustainable changes:

- Follow the 80/20 rule wherein you eat healthily 80% of the time and allow yourself leeway for indulgences the remaining 20%.

- Find healthy alternatives for your favorite snacks.

- Cook more meals at home which can help control what goes into your food.

- Exercise regularly; staying physically active can help regulate your appetite and make you more mindful of your body's needs.

11.4. Patience and Forgiveness: Your Lifelong Companions

Nobody's perfect, and expecting perfection from yourself in maintaining a balanced life can lead to disappointment and unnecessary pressure. Embrace patience and forgiveness as invaluable tools to deal with failures.

Practicing patience allows you to understand that lifestyle changes might take more time than you initially imagined. Forgiving yourself for slips not only eases the guilt but also empowers you to pick up where you left and keep moving forward.

11.5. Cultivating a Supportive Environment

The role of a supportive environment and social network in reinforcing good eating habits cannot be overstated. Here's how to cultivate such an environment:

- Surround yourself with like-minded individuals committed to leading a healthy lifestyle.

- Engage in activities that promote wellness.

- Leverage the power of digital communities. Join online health and wellness groups to keep yourself motivated and accountable.

As you assimilate these practices into your everyday life, remember that sustainability and balance are key factors in maintaining this newfound freedom. The art of food freedom isn't about severe restrictions, but more about flexibility, awareness, and kindness towards oneself. Enjoy the journey and remember, you're doing incredibly well, one step at a time.